Body Prayers:
Finding Body Peace

1

Other Books by Rebecca Radcliffe

Enlightened Eating: Understanding and Changing Your Relationship with Food

Dance Naked In Your Living Room: Handling Stress & Finding Joy

Hot Flashes, Chocolate Sauce, & Rippled Thighs: Women's Wisdom, Wellness, Self-Acceptance & Joy

About To Burst: Handling Stress & Ending Violence— A Message for Youth

Dedication:

Body Prayers™ is dedicated to the strength of the feminine and the miracle of women's lives. The power of the feminine to nurture and connect is exactly what the world needs to solve many of the problems we face in the coming years. It is time that we as women apply our gifts toward ourselves to develop greater self-acceptance and the confidence to pursue our dreams. Together, we can promote tolerance of all sorts—including an appreciation of different body sizes and shapes.

Address All Inquiries to Publisher:
EASE™ Publications
P.O. Box 8032
Minneapolis, Minnesota, 55408-0032 USA
1-800-470-4769/www.livingtogrow.com

Manufactured in the United States of America

Alternative Cataloguing-In-Publication Data

Radcliffe, Rebecca
        Body prayers™: finding body peace--a journey of self acceptance. Minneapolis, MN: EASE, copyright 2004.

        1. Body image. 2. Women's self-esteem 3. Eating issues--body hatred. 4. Self-help psychology.
        I. Title. II. Title: Body prayers™. III. Title: Finding body peace--a journey of self acceptance. IV. EASE.

    ISBN 0-9636607-2-1

    Library of Congress Number 98-094897

BODY PRAYERS:

Finding Body Peace

by rebecca radcliffe

a journey of self-acceptance

EASE™ Publications, P.O. Box 8032, Minneapolis, Minnesota, 55408-0032 USA
Design & cover art by Beth Ruggles

Part 1:

The Vision:
One World,
Many Sizes

Dear Friends:

Body Prayers™ is for all females who learned to dislike the natural curves and shapes of their bodies. Very few of us can stand naked in front of a mirror and accept what we see.

Instead, we see curves and rolls that we wish would go away. Our hearts sink when we think how many times we've tried to diet or exercise those inches away.

We blame ourselves and our lack of will-power. We sigh with resignation as we finish getting dressed to go out into the world and do our day. It undermines our confidence to follow our dreams. We think, *"How can we better our world when we can't even lose five pounds?"*

These are the signs of body hatred. There are millions of women of all ages who are affected by body dissatisfaction. It is a modern affliction that developed in the early 1960's when

Twiggy hit the scene with an oddly thin and wispy figure.

Our society's obsession with thinness has continued to grow to the point that it has changed our thinking about what is beautiful and undermined women's self-esteem.

Sadly, it has played a major role in the development of the eating disorders, over-eating, binging, and depression that affect countless women.

Any female who has played with Barbie, looked at fashion magazines, or watched television broadcasts and movies since the early 1960's, is infected with the wide-spread social belief that thin is the only shape that is beautiful.

Our natural shapes and sizes do not match the media images we see. We cannot match these ultra-thin shapes without becoming anorexic or bulimic. We cannot have large breasts on thin bodies without surgery. We cannot have the perfect skin and smooth body lines we see in air-brushed and computer-augmented advertisements.

Yet we still compare ourselves each and every day to the images in the media. We measure ourselves against the women we see in magazines, on television, on the streets, and around us everyday. We feel straddled with thicker, rounder, less attractive figures.

Media messages tell us that thin women find love and get promoted at the office. A skinny body is the ticket. Our unruly bodies do not measure up. Our lives will not be as "full."

It is time to change this destructive view of women's bodies. Skinny images have created far too much depression, low self-esteem, and diet-related health problems among women of all ages. We need to work together to create more tolerance so that body discrimination will no longer hold women back or erode their confidence.

As we bring about a new climate of body acceptance and size tolerance, women will be free to focus on shaping better lives for themselves and bettering the world. No longer will so much time, energy, and money be channeled into worrying about appearances.

A shift to appreciating body diversity can only happen when women lead the way. Media images will change only when women question and reject what they see.

Body Prayers™ is a tool to help you on that journey of questioning and rebirth. It will help you gently explore and hopefully change your feelings about your body.

Tolerance must begin with each of us individually. We can grow to accept ourselves and our unique body shape as well as the body shapes of the women we know and love.

Together and over time, we can create a different world for ourselves, our daughters, and all women to come.

Warmly,

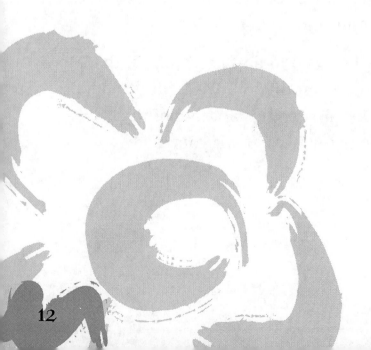

Part 2

The Journey:
Finding
Body Peace

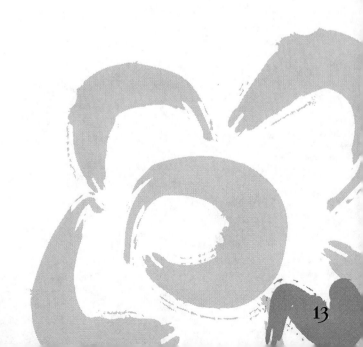

Today, I gently begin. I am looking for a place of peace, a way to find acceptance within.

I seek to discover and appreciate your wonder instead of criticizing every line and curve.

I am too bruised and confused to know what's true anymore. So I must listen from my heart.

Help me find the way, my deepest soul.

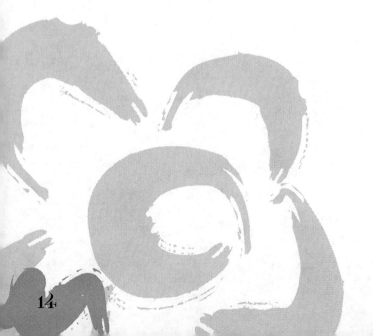

Years of mirrors and magazines have smashed my hope of feeling beautiful, soft, round. I cringe when I see my body pushing out the edges of my clothing. Those curves push away love. They smother me and choke off my dreams. Today, I put away those magazines and seek a new mirror in which to more clearly see who I am.

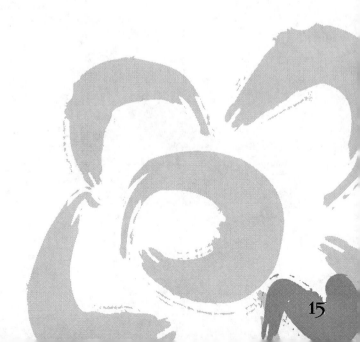

I feel the hatred start again whenever I notice the tightness of my waistband or how the folds of my body stack one on top of another. I vow again and again to chase them away with every ounce of strength I can muster. But it is never enough. I am never enough. The sorrow of this thinking is easily enough to drown me.

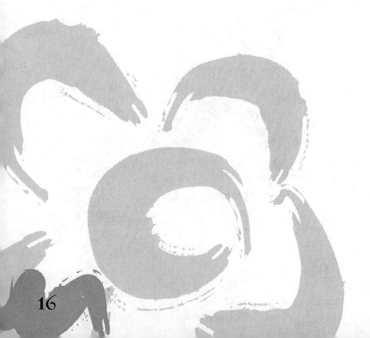

Approximately 7 million women and 1 million men are afflicted with an eating disorder.[4]

I watch others and wonder if their bodies seem as painful to them as mine is to me. Do they worry when their hunger starts? Do they dread the morning, the scale, the closet, the mirror, the cupboards, the refrigerator? Do they see beauty or do they cringe when they glimpse themselves in windows or vanities? Do they hate magazines in checkout-lanes that promise a perfect body this time? I must be crazy to seek peace in a tiny-sized reality. I really want a world of magnificent, giant-sized possibilities.

Years of looking at food-restricted, saline-breasted, workout-pounded, made-over, surgically-constructed, and computer-enhanced media images defeat me utterly. Gone are tribal memories of abundance and power in female girth. Gone is respect of femininity as equal. Giving birth is no longer a miracle. Numbers and lines. Thinness and power. Profit and greed. These have replaced being connected. Connection—to others and the earth—used to be necessary for survival. It was worthy of reverence and great respect. No longer. This must change.

I carry the struggle and stress of my life in this very body which I judge so harshly. My body carries me; it suffers my intake of fast food, no sleep, high stress, and little joy. I never worry if it will be there the next day or if it will desert me on a whim. It remains faithful and constant. I take it for granted, and I apologize. This is no way to conduct or value a relationship.

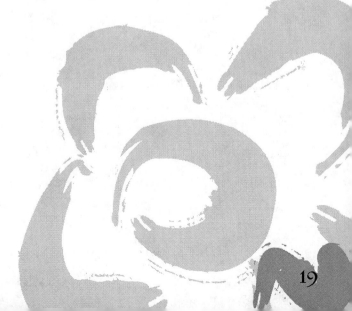

19

Anorexia nervosa affects approximately 1% of adolescent girls. Bulimia nervosa affects approximately 2-3 %.[7]

There are weeds in my soul—I can feel them choking off the light. They are hard to control, and make my body uncomfortable, full, stuffed with an uneasiness. How nerve-racking! So I find myself creeping toward the kitchen, breaking every promise, failing once again to stem the bulging tide of my body. The power of food seduces me. I munch away, forgetting the weeds, forgetting my soul.

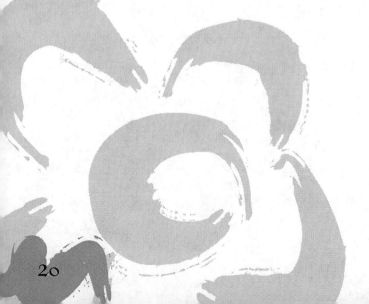

They say the body is a temple. I wonder if mine could be. Temples are holy; the way I eat and live isn't holy. Temples are gorgeous and inspiring; I don't feel inspiring and definitely not gorgeous. Temples are close to God, and I don't have the answers. But I am very good at cleaning things, and I can love. Perhaps a bit of appreciation and elbow grease will build a whole new structure.

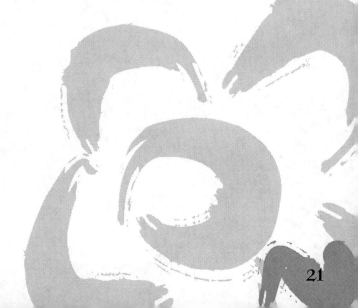

I am lost in the piles of garbage within me. Darkness has swallowed all but the tiniest light. My hope is faltering. Will I ever find a way through? Shovels, back-hoes, dump trucks. . .nothing would be enough for the piles stuck and stuffed inside me. Every big and little hurt of mine is crammed in here. Cementing into pounds of tension, pain, and depression—they beg for release. So do I. I want to run straight to my refrigerator, but I take the next step instead. I choose to grow.

I lose patience some days and would rather forget about changing. Nothing seems to change very fast. I could even be going backward—how would I know? No one has ever lived in a world of body peace. I suspect it will feel as if a hundred pounds were lifted from my body when I get there. Meanwhile, I focus on the work in front of me and take another step.

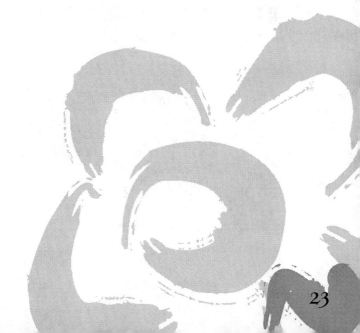

I want to feel new and lovely, round and secure, joyful and intrigued by my life. It can start in my body. Then I'd have the security to do anything. Good things in my day could also swirl back to help me feel better in my body. Something new is growing. I am onto something. My soul feels hopeful. We are adventuring, exploring, and experimenting together. It feels good to be on the move.

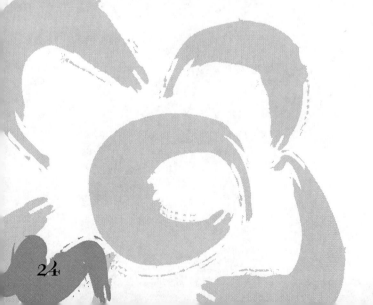

Of 2,000 black women responding to a non-culturally sensitive survey, 71.5% felt preoccupied with the desire to be thinner and an equal number were terrified of being overweight.[12]

I congratulate myself for continuing. There are days I'd rather give up. Sometimes, I'd rather scream ragefully. Other days, I blame everyone else for mucking things up. But only I can set this life adrift into a new pattern. So I take a deep breath, swallow hard, give myself a word of encouragement, and take yet another step. How many will it take to get there?

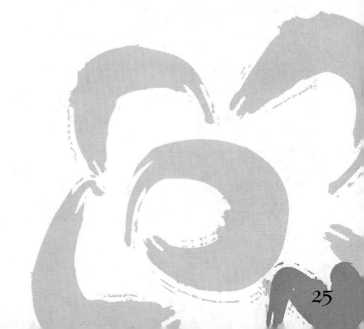

Sometimes it's the wind that comforts me. I feel it on my face and in my hair. It holds me, shakes me, and even pushes me forward when I resist. Morning birds call me to keep trying, And the scent of rain brings mystery. Guidance on this difficult journey often shows up in someone's laugh or offhand comment, a song's lyric, or a coincidence. Funny thing, how learning goes.

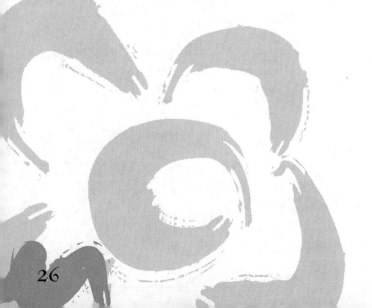

I gently coax myself forward little by little. I am tired of the harassment, blame, belittlement, and shame I level at myself. I rebel against this harshness. No, I wish to be kind. What do I want? What do I need? What a relief to be learning respect for my body. It's sad that it's taken so long.

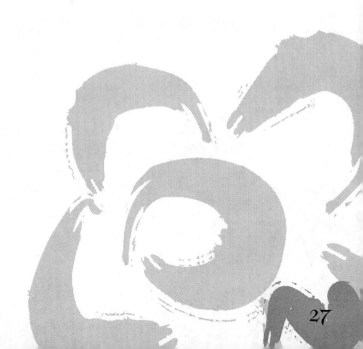

27

I am practicing being a good provider. I give my body the sleep it needs, good water to drink, clean air to breathe, supportive friends to be with, healthy foods for fuel, interesting work to engage me, good activity to spark my joy, renewing quiet, and time to reflect. This is the new shape of my life. I am healing. I am learning to be well. I care for the body that carries me. This way, we both thrive.

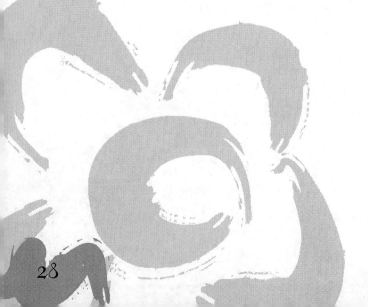

Each step is so blasted small! Am I really going anywhere? I hate all the effort one tiny change takes. Everyday I push. No giving up. There are signs of hope. I question the advertiser for using the skinny model instead of freaking about my size. I don't panic at every hunger pang. Now clothes that don't honor me or my body are gone. No more uncomfortable, ugly, seductive, or "not me" stuff anymore. I choose comfort, colors, self-expression, and joy for my life.

I'm wistful sometimes when I see skinny, bone-thin shapes. These are the bodies that everyone watches and envies. My body has never cooperated. I have always felt ugly. My legs aren't straight. My waist is wrong. My face is ordinary, plain. Everything bulges. Pretty, attractive, beautiful…these are foreign to me. If beauty radiates from within, don't the seeds of belief first have to be planted? Do these seeds even exist? Where do I find them?

Today my body pushed really hard. It got up early, exercised, worked hard all day, handled stress and deadlines, took me home, did chores, and stayed up late without protest. Day after day, it's the same. No wonder it gets tired, sick, discouraged, depressed. This is no way to live. My body never gets a chance to refuel. One day, it might not be able to bounce back. I better think about this now.

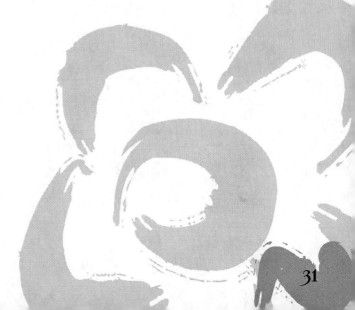

This tummy, these thighs, and this full rear end have haunted me for years. They have plagued me in fitting rooms, embarrassed me on dates, discouraged me from trying new things, and depleted my self-confidence. They hold the power to ruin my life! They stop me from flirting, getting jobs, and believing I'll ever be loved. I hate these curves. Why, oh, why can't I be flat, tall, thin, and wonderful?

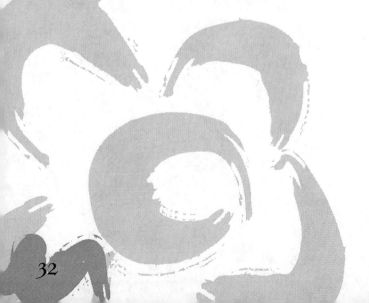

One hundred percent of formerly fat people would rather be deaf, dyslexic, diabetic, or have bad acne or heart disease than be obese again. 91% would rather have a leg amputated.[20]

Maybe it's not the curves. Maybe it's me. Maybe it's the messages I've heard. The TV tells me certain cereals will get me thin. They don't work for me. I must have a problem. Others tell me I'll look good in my jeans in only five days. But my body never changes that fast. Is there something wrong with me, or is someone lying to make a buck?

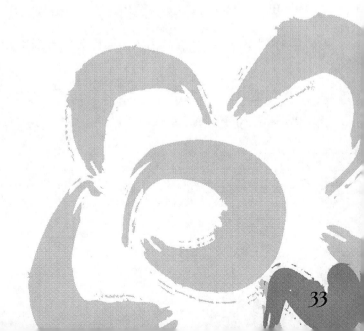

How dare you tell me your perfume will make me more genuine! How dare you ask me to pay you to starve myself! How dare you hurt young girls and women by telling them they're ugly when they're round! How dare you tell me using your toothpaste will bring me love? We're strong, feisty, beautiful, capable, gifted, talented, smart, dedicated, and committed women. We're not stupid. Shame on you for seducing us into spending hours in our closets, the gym, or in front of the mirror. We should be working hard to better ourselves and the world!

During my lifetime, I hope our society will come to appreciate that bodies come in all different sizes and shapes. Our ancestors spawned us from bodies that endured hardship and pain, disease and storm, hunger and war. Today, we go to any store and find plenty of food. Our bodies still protect us from starving even when we wish they'd let us lose a few pounds. Someday, we may still be grateful for this ability to endure.

I love to watch all of the wonderful female bodies in my locker room. Each is so amazingly different from another. All are beautiful. The young adolescent bodies and the aging pendulant bodies both have their stories. The tight and trim, and the round and the ample. Bodies carry women through their journeys. They support, nurture, give birth, endure, move, age, and grow in a most marvelous way. Watching these beautiful shapes reminds me that size does not equal beauty.

I pray to love this body as it is, to accept the size that I am, and move on to more important things. If only I was truly free to do that. I'd have to be able to see the television, movies, and magazines without comparing myself to their skinny images. I'd have to feel beautiful as I move through my days. I'd have to know that my shape and size do not affect my ability to be who I am. I'd have to focus on improving my life and the world instead changing my body. This is the dream.

> Disney's Pocahontas is a woman we all know well...whose unlikely shape is found on thousands of [truckers] mud flaps. Whose waist is so small she cannot have any internal organs.[25]

When I have moments where my body size or shape doesn't matter, it's wonderful. The days I am with friends and forget to rank order them all by size inside my head are precious. The times I forget the shape of my body and just have fun are quite delicious. The times I laugh hard and forget my self-conscious feelings about my body heal me deeply. Even a few moments like this teach me what is possible.

My fits of anger at my body hurt the most. I pound through my exercise, ready to kill any impulse to eat or gain. My shape disgusts me. Self-hatred courses through me and rages in my head. 'Why can't you get it together? Why are you so lazy, stupid, weak, ugly? Why did you break your promise to do better?' I wear myself down until I'm broken, hopeless, and feeling rotten. I know raging at myself is disheartening, but who else is there?

Then I remember—a perfect body isn't the answer.

Body Dysmorphic Disorder—an obsessive concern with the size or shape of one or more body parts—afflicts an estimated 5 million Americans.[27]

My body feelings are very old. I remember getting messages very early that never stopped: chiding from a parent, teasing from a sibling, name-calling on the playground, rude comments from a visitor or stranger, harsh judgement from a physician, shaming from a lover, whispers at work. There were the hours playing with Barbie dolls, inspections of my emerging body, and the awkward, ugly feelings that took shape as my body developed out of control. No wonder body hatred grows so deep and mean.

As young girls, we bud like roses with enthusiasm and wonder. Our capacity to give and love does the world great good if it grows without bruising. Too often, this tenderness tempts harsh souls who grab, caress, take, and destroy. Weeping, shaking, and deeply scarred, we have to cope and go on, usually in silence and without support. When we don't hold rapists, drunk drivers, corporate raiders, and bullies of all sorts accountable, we perpetuate this brutality.

41

The vital statistics of today's mannequins are so extreme that any woman actually shaped in such a way would have too little body fat to menstruate.[29]

I got it loud and clear: bodies count. I see other girls and women dressing skimpily, waggling their hips, skinnying down, and getting breast implants to be desirable. I have to decide—do I 'put out' or not? Do I make myself look right for someone else to enjoy, or do I create my own unique self to present to the world? The skinny bodies we're supposed to want can be dangerous.

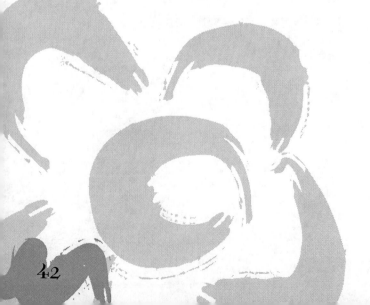

In our society today, female athletes are increasingly at risk for the "Female Athletic Triad:" disordered eating, amenorrhea (lack of menstruation), and osteoporosis (bone weakening).[30]

I see how thinness opens doors. It turns heads. It entices, intrigues, turns on, and teases people with status, looks, money, and fame. But thinness can't keep away pain. Break-ups, loneliness, fear, vulnerability, job loss, and money troubles can happen anyway. Does being thin give me real strength? Does it help me defend myself when under attack? Does it give me the size and endurance I need to cope with a challenging world?

For black girls, beauty is taking what one has and using it well. Weight is not the issue, it's how one moves. And beauty doesn't end at 25: mothers and grandmothers are called beautiful, too.[31]

I sometimes wonder if women were seen for their creativity and abilities instead of for their looks, wouldn't the world be an incredibly different place? I wouldn't worry as much about what I put on in the morning. I wouldn't think as much about the numbers on the scale. I wouldn't obsess about the bulge under my jeans. I could celebrate instead the new ideas I had each day and the lessons I learned. I would value everything that made me smarter and more capable. Don't we all deserve this?

I pray today for self-love, for my own tolerance of who I am. I pray today that I dare express some of my real thoughts and feelings and move in the direction of my dreams. I pray today that I will be released from my self doubts a little bit more each day. I pray that I can help shape our culture so that women behind me will find a more welcoming world. I pray today that I find other women and men who will protest these judgements and work together to make this a more sacred world.

If only more men were gentle as well as strong. If only more men were turned on by caring as well as chemistry. If only more men considered relationships with themselves, their families, the world, and the planet as good investments. If only more men would teach their sons to protect instead of conquer. If only more men would embrace women as equals instead of defending their right to the top of the heap. If only more men would create a world in which their daughters could soar. These would be men with grace.

Changing my body is not as simple as deciding to eat less or differently. It is not about food much at all. It is about my attitudes, the world in which we live, the restraints put on women's lives, the decisions women must make in response to these limits. This world is changing, and women are leading the way. We can no longer be molded into cute little playmates that keep a neat house. It's not enough. My body tells me I am strong and capable, and I am thrilled to discover all that I can become.

I hope I have the courage to invent myself in this new way. If I leave behind what society taught me about being acceptable, then I won't have many role models. Only a few leaders, authors, and thinkers who refuse to fit quietly into the world will illuminate the way. Me, I am no leader or great thinker. I am scared of being left out. I don't want to be alone. But an empty life of appearances and following everyone's rules will kill me, too. Courage is being willing to just to take another step.

My soul is delighted when I choose to nurture myself rather than to complain about my body size. When I choose to grow instead of worrying about calories, my inner self cheers. When I express my thoughts and feelings rather than hiding my true self, my confidence expands. I wish I could have learned this in school. I wish someone could have coached me into becoming a strong woman instead of praising my ability to be good, sweet, kind, and adaptable. Well, better now than never.

No one will know what to make of me now. This journey has me excited about finding myself and what I really like. I'm taking better care of myself, making sure my life is balanced, and making plans for even more changes. Frankly, it's unnerving some of my friends and family. They'd rather have the old, comfortable me. That wasn't me; I was just pretending to make them happy. But I wasn't happy. Now I have a real chance to create a life that suits me.

And what about my body? What about all of these curves? Well, maybe they'll change someday. Maybe my body is where it likes to be. Maybe it's covering up old pain that I'll discover and release along the way. I don't know yet. But my plans to match the magazine pages don't seem as important as discovering my dreams. My body size has nothing to do with expressing myself or developing a career or creative outlet. My visions and attitudes are much more important. Let's see where my dreams take me.

Today, I promise to take care of you, my body, treat you gently, and give you what you need. I can't make this journey without you, so you are my first priority. You will get nourishing food, good sun and air, time outside, plenty of rest, stimulating activities, and time to move. I am grateful for your health and strength. I take my responsibility of keeping you on a healthy path seriously. I make my choices with your energy and vitality in mind. Thank you for all you do for me.

When discouragement comes, my load seems too heavy and the climb too impossible. My dreams seem silly and impossible. Someone's criticism hit too hard, right when I was most vulnerable. Why would they understand? They don't seem to mind the world as it is. But I do. I want my life to be different. I want the world to be more fair to me and those of my shape. I want women to have a million chances to succeed at anything they want. I hope I feel better tomorrow.

After a storm, the air clears. Thank goodness. That darkness, the crashing all around, the debris flying is more than frightening. But God sends the sun back out, paints the sky blue again, and makes the air so fresh it seems like heaven. That's when I believe it's possible to go on. I feel whipped, wiped out, wrung weak, but slowly, slowly things return to normal. My confidence returns, and I continue journeying into my new life. Storms and criticism always exist, even when we don't choose to change.

Here is my dream: friend to friend, mother to daughter, co-worker to colleague, neighbor to neighbor, stranger to stranger, women together can question the narrow standards of beauty and size. I hope we stop comparing ourselves to others and stop criticizing each other. I fantasize that we hear praise for our ideas and create an environment where our talents can thrive. Since women still largely raise the children, I believe we can be a strong influence in the world to come. Our voices make a difference if we use them.

The silence I learned as a girl chokes me most when I'm hurt or angry. I was taught not to rock the boat. Well, the waters inside me are churning anyway, and my boat is rocking! My silence keeps the secrets hidden, keeps the pain from healing, keeps changes from happening. I hate for others to reject my ideas, to think I'm too brash or angry, to judge me as intolerant or selfish. I'm just being honest. Truth hurts, but so does the lie of swallowing our words.

Can the world can change? Absolutely! Do I worry about this when I see so much stupidity everywhere? Yes. Is it still worth the effort to make a difference? Without question. I have only one opportunity to live this lifetime. I cannot waste it. Being complacent would be my biggest crime against life. I am here to become wiser, deepen my heart, and offer what I can. If nothing else, my own life improves as I grow. And I have more to give. So I keep going in spite of where the world is headed.

The effect of my new choices are becoming
noticeable to me. When I eat fresh, whole
foods, I have more strength and less cravings.
When I take time to sleep, I feel more rested
and positive. When I exercise and move, I feel
more grounded in my body and better able to
cope. Time with friends is good for my heart.
A good book stimulates my mind. Better work
makes me happier indeed. Can I tell things are
happening? Definitely!

Now when I look in the mirror, I see the woman I am and want to be. Sometimes, she is tired and confused, but she tries awfully hard. I am proud of that. Can I criticize the roundness of her belly when together, we are taking on such big life changes? I still wish for it to be flatter, but it doesn't matter as much anymore. My body is healthier with these changes, and my clothes are fitting differently.

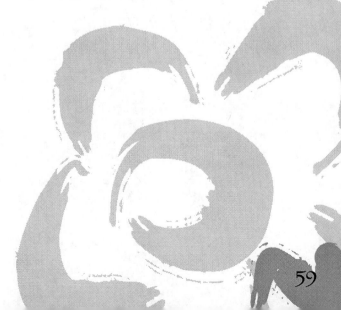

I am beginning to walk in a new kind of power. It is the power of being me. I do not have to pretend to be happy. I do not have to be a creep. I just have the simple joy from being more myself than ever before. This wonderful sensation helps get me through bad moods and tough times. Feeling this feminine power of endurance is a delight. It has nothing to do with my body looking like the images in the media. It has everything to do with my life matching the needs of my soul more closely.

Today I celebrate my changes. I give myself credit. I am proud of the fact that I dare swim upstream. I am not accepting the messages that I am only as good as I am thin. No, I am creative and courageous for being willing to question and grow. I reject the simplistic notion that women should spend lots of time shaping and decorating themselves to appeal to others. This is my life, and I want it to appeal to me.

I still work hard to reject the "skinniness is everything" message. I don't buy women's magazines. I question the ads that try to convince me to eat or buy something. In conversation, I don't let obnoxious comments about women's bodies slide by. I praise myself for my many efforts to become a better person rather than focusing on my shape or size. But I'd rather be free altogether and have size not be an issue for women.

In a study of 48 women ages 25-67, those who fulfilled their early dreams were overwhelmingly satisfied with their life even when success came late; those who had not tried, regretted it.[50]

I wonder if it is possible for all women to reject these images strongly enough to make a difference? Alone, my voice feels small and weak in this fight. I need others to question, too. I will feel more sane, less alone. I know most women hate how society judges female bodies. We're just afraid to admit it and be seen as different.

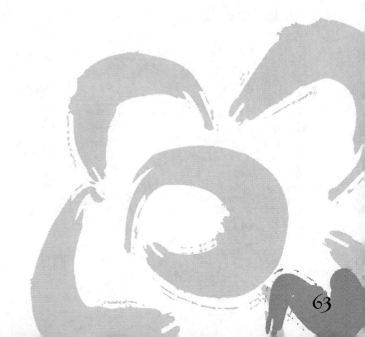

I cringe to think that if I stay quiet, the next batch of young women will suffer just as I have. Unless we protest, the obsession will go on. Too many people like women weak, distracted by our appearances, focused on getting skinny instead of tackling the real problems in the world. Women are incredibly powerful. They are the glue of most families, and could change the world radically if their creative energy was fully unleashed. No wonder those in control would rather have us dieting.

I am beginning to see myself as strong and capable, a creature of talent. I used to see only body parts out of control...legs, breasts, hips, and thighs that would not behave. I was only as good as my body, and that failed to measure up. Depression ate away my hopes and dreams. How could I do anyone or anything any good in such an imperfect form? There is something really wrong with a world that does this to women.

65

It worries me that little girls are counting the calories in french fries, drinking liquid shakes, and staying away from fattening foods. They look at their bodies in the mirror and call themselves fat…just like their moms and sisters do. Parents see their babies' chubby little bodies and water down their juice. Hasn't this gone too far? We have gotten NUTS about skinny bodies. And everyone who isn't thin has gotten the message: **YOU ARE NOT OK.** I'm sending one back: **YES I AM. WHO ARE YOU TO TELL ME OTHERWISE?**

When I look at trees, I see how different each one is. There are tall ones, short ones, elegant column trees, bushy round trees, crooked trees, and perfectly straight trees. Is one shape more beautiful than another? Am I to judge one as best? Nature creates variety for a reason. Diversity makes it stronger and better at survival. When I try to fit one idea of perfection, my creativity dies, too,

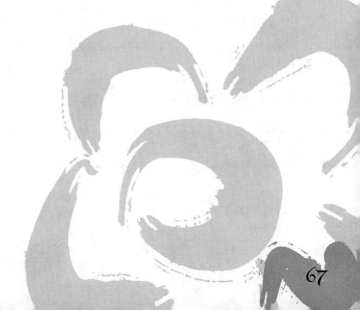

I have a growing kindness toward other people's bodies. After all, if I want to be accepted as I am, then I must learn to see large and small, fit and unfit, and classically attractive and unattractive bodies as beautiful. I believe this in principle…but overcoming years of conditioning takes more effort than I imagined. Too often, my first judgement of other bodies comes through society's glasses. I catch myself labeling people as "fat" or "ugly" or "different." I stop myself, shake my head clear of these narrow boxes, and then affirm the right of everyone to be as they are.

I feel bombarded by comments about women's bodies these days. Maybe it's just my growing sensitivity to the subject. I hear women in bathrooms, on talk shows, in sitcoms, on news programs, even in books and magazine headlines—everywhere women talk about their discomfort with their bodies and their envy of those who fit society's expectations. All I have to do is tune in. We are obsessed with thinness.

When I get myself up and out to walk, bike, swim, run, dance, swing, or do an aerobics class, I am delighted with how it makes me feel. Fresh air and blood race through me. I feel stronger and more appreciative of my body. I am alive and ready to do my day. This body is made for moving, but I did not know it until recently. It was easier to sit. It took effort to "work out." I was too busy. I got stuck, enlarged, soft. Learning to move has changed my energy, well-being, and body forever.

Hopping between my covers and sinking in to sleep after a busy day is such a treat. The hard part is getting to bed early enough to feel completely rested before the demands of the next morning. When I bound out of bed eager for the day, then I know I've gotten enough sleep. Too often, it's a chore to get up. I cut corners on sleep—but I'm only cheating myself. Too little dream time. Too little time for dreams work out the stress. How can I expect joy from life if I am all wrung out with fatigue? How can my body keep going?

When I'm really drained, my body craves energy. I roam through cupboards trying to find something satisfying—a "pick-me-up." Chocolate, colas, coffee, sugar-filled goodies, yummy pastas and breadstuffs: these work best. But they don't stop the cravings. Stuffing in empty calories is no way to keep the fires burning. Maybe I'm getting a different kind of signal. Maybe my body wants me to rest well and eat healthy (fats, protein, fruits, vegies, whole grains) in the first place. I need to listen better.

When I'm having fun...when I am doing things that interest me...when I connect with people I like, my body seems happiest. I stay healthier, have more energy, feel better about myself, and am more optimistic. The size of my waistline doesn't seem to top the list of critical issues if I am doing good stuff. This is the challenge: how can I get and keep the flow of friendly and creative energy moving in my life? I am not here just to get by. That is too empty. I want quality time while I am here on earth.

Twenty-five years ago, the secret subject of women was sex. Today it's food.[61]

If only I dare try the dreams of my life—
designing clothes; painting murals; starting a
business; becoming independent; writing songs;
learning to take pictures; doing stand-up
comedy; traveling cross country; going on a
retreat. Will I ever do any of them? Not if I
stay stuck in this routine. Not if I get
depressed every evening. Not by believing I
am not smart or brave enough. To begin takes
one step: one class, one poem, one drawing,
or one idea. The joy of even one creative step
can make my heart soar.

My body needs quiet time, down time, connecting time. Then I can let the pain of the day empty out. I can hear the needs of my body, of my heart, of my soul. Otherwise, life chatters and roars around me, and my inner self gets lost. I cherish the moments of sitting in my favorite chair, of swinging in the back-yard, of soaking in a hot scented tub. The lost and lonely parts of me begin to reassemble again the more time I spend connecting with myself.

This question of what is sacred, of what makes life spiritual keeps cycling back around for me to deal with. The crazy spin of life events and achievement is not enough to keep me happy. No lottery ticket or triple dark chocolate truffle cake, perfect career, or great romance is going to fill the deepest parts of me. There must be something more to this stay on earth. What is my purpose? Of what am I part? Where do I go next? I seek for deeper answers that can fill my life and quiet my heart.

My body is becoming more important and holy to me. It needs to be treated with dignity, reverence, and great care. This is a huge shift for me. Before, I trudged through each day, pushing and demanding my body follow any pace I set, healthy or not. I assumed it would just keep chugging. But what if I am really destined to live 150 or 200 years (as experts are beginning to say)? Could I keep up this unhealthy pace and routine that long? No way. My body would fail before that.

My animals teach me how to unwind. They sleep an awful lot. They love to play. They are ready for a quick game or outdoors scamper at a moment's notice. They watch birds, squirrels, leaves, and passing traffic to keep themselves interested. They know who their friends are and keep close. They sniff, stretch, scratch, and clean themselves regularly. They eat when they are hungry, and don't need fancy diets. There are important clues here for me!

I'm making a list of ways to care for myself and my body. It seems silly, but I never learned to make caring for myself a priority. I just tense up, grab something to eat, feel crummy, take a deep breath, and plow forward 'til the cycle repeats itself. My body has taken the brunt of the stress and what I stuff into it to unwind. I am learning to turn on music, do yoga, meditate, scream in a pillow, write in a journal, pull weeds, water the plants—there are a hundred ways to unwind the stress that grips my day.

What fun! I am throwing things away. Anything that holds a bad memory goes. Clothes that don't fit me are goners! Decorations or furnishings I don't like anymore get donated along with books and stuff that just collect dust. I am keeping only what I love. When I surround myself with things that bring me contentment, the flow of joy in my life increases. Everything I've physically and emotionally outgrown, I release from my life. This makes space for new and wonderful things to come.

In one study, children fed a low-fat, complex carbohydrate, lean meat diet, received only 60% of required calories without the 25-37% fat calories needed and suffered weight/height loss.[68]

Choosing how I live each day is a sacred act. I value the time and the body I've been given. Each choice I make reflects how I feel about myself and this gift of earthly time. If I squander my days and make poor choices that eventually rob me of energy or health, then I do not honor the opportunity to heal both my life and the world. I affect others, whatever my choices. So I try to live with quality. My contribution will be as positive as I know how to make it whether the ripples I make are small or big.

"Failure to thrive" in infants and children is usually a result of illness, poverty, or neglect. It is a new and growing phenomenon among middle-class, health-conscious parents.[69]

What do I do with my anger when it boils over? When I explode, I don't care how hateful or horrible I am to my body. I say the meanest things. I am rude on the roads. I burst, shatter, bust, into a million painful, slamming, destructive pieces. I can't think, I don't care, I don't know what to do. If I could get junk out before I reach the breaking point, it'd be much better. We're supposed to be so nice, so I pretend I'm OK. Sometimes, when I feel really nasty inside, but I think I've got it under control, it bursts out onto someone else before they have a clue that something is wrong. What a mess.

Loving my body means making new choices all the way around. It's more work than I imagined. I thought I could blame it all on the media. It is a huge part of the problem, but being good to myself involves much more than getting rid of skinny pictures. Loving myself means accepting me as I am. It means trying to listen and respect my needs. It means give and take and compromise. It means daring to dream. Daring to live. And choosing to live with meaning and quality.

With every breath, I breathe in new life. I breathe in a new way of seeing myself. I breathe in a gentle tendril of love for my evolving life. With every release of my breath, I breathe out the old, the outgrown, the useless, the destructive messages I held onto too long. I let go of hurt, pain, and self-destruction. I take in renewal. I let out hopelessness. I affirm new life, and I let go of fears and limiting beliefs. I am renewed each day, each moment, with each breath.

The presence of food issues often causes an internal tension for other women as they ask: *who is eating less? who is working out more? who is the fattest and thinnest of the group?*[72]

Laying on the floor, I close my eyes and relax my body from my head through my face, neck, torso, and legs, and on to my toes. I thank each part for doing its job of carrying me. I thank the inner parts of me for breathing, digesting, filtering, healing, building, eliminating, and aerating so I can live with vitality. I notice small pains and promise to search out ways to heal. Noticing my needs, I promise to live with greater balance. I fill my body with golden light, putting extra on sore spots. When ready, I gently get up.

I see more coincidences…more gifts that come my way as I flow into this growth. A friend is willing to talk about something painful and resolve it. A chance to vacation in a wonderful place occurs when I least expect it. A thought crosses my mind and turns into a whole new way of thinking about things. A contact for a new job comes into my life just when I could use it. There are tiny miracles here each and every day. Learning to recognize and be grateful for them is part of my task.

The gift of connection with a friend or love warms my heart and brings hope to my life. I do not take love of any sort for granted; it is too easy to grow apart. I have lost friends due to distance, job changes, new cities, new interests, misunderstandings, and jealousies. Luckily, new friends came to me again from different jobs, schooling, relationships, neighborhoods, meetings, etc. I nurture and protect them, for their interest in me and loving reflection nourishes my soul.

Being totally honest with myself about my body isn't easy. Neither is being honest with my friends when I hurt. Is there a parallel here? What am I hiding? What don't I want to admit? What am I afraid of losing? I do not want to rock the boat. I don't want to feel all my pain. I don't want to lose the approval of those I care about. So I just shut up. When my reality is less than pretty, I often pretend I'm alright. Then people can't see the whole me. Could I dare share more? Will they stay?

> Demand feeding, a strategy involving not putting any foods in a bad or taboo category and eating whenever one is hungry, may be the "cure" for body hatred.[76]

Standing naked in my truth is very hard. I panic when I realize what others must think of me. I am different. I no longer pursue body perfection as my goal in life. I have begun to question. I think about my dreams. I am willing to go down a different path. That scares some people way too much. Will I be utterly alone on this journey? I can no longer accept that my body is wrong or ugly. I refuse to accept that I cannot live my dream. I must grow past society's limits for women. I want to dance my own dance.

I stand in front of my mirror today without cringing. My body is just a body. It's job is to breathe, carry me, create energy, and be strong. It's not to tease, seduce, attract, or tantalize. The world cannot know whether I'm a good, creative, interesting, or smart person from judging my body. So I accept what I see. It still doesn't match the ads. But I love my body for sticking by me in spite of my abuse. It remains loyal, beautiful, and blossoming under my new and gentler regime of self-care.

Appearance anxiety is highest among middle-class women of means who cannot tolerate "letting themselves go" for fear of abandonment, loneliness, and dependency.[78]

I still don't have the ideal body, but I'm willing to move on from here. In a perfect world, I'd change my shape or change all advertisements. Since I cannot do either, I'll be content with focusing on more important issues. It's time to get on with my dreams. Why should the shape of my body take so much focus? No more calories counting. No more food plans. No more unhappy workouts. I am declaring a truce. I'm no longer at war with my body. We are learning to peacefully coexist. Thank goodness.

Learning to be a peaceful partner with my body is such a delight. I am becoming free of my old self-hatred. Hating my body took more energy and brought me down a lot more than I realized. My life journey has little to do with body size. Rather, it has been about courage, the willingness to dream, being emotionally honest, and growing as much as I can. I can do that thin or fat, tall or short, big or little, young or old. I am here to dream, not to get thin.

This new perspective is so different! Some days I am scared so deeply I'm afraid I might cave in and give up. But I put one foot forward and take another little step. Before long, I feel the difference. I've moved into a new phase. I see the change. I become energized, open, and intrigued by things again. Thank goodness I am no longer strangled by one definition of perfection. I am thrilled to learn and watch my life blossom. Here I come!

Body tolerance takes continued effort. I go along fine accepting myself when suddenly, I see a skinny person being kissed. My heart cringes, and I worry that I am on the wrong path. That I'll miss out on love and success because my body will never be thin. Then I find my center and get my thinking on straight: just because things look perfect doesn't mean they are. More importantly, what are my goals? What do I want for my life? I wish the thin person well, and then turn my focus back on my own growth and well-being.

I've been careful not to pass this craziness down to my daughter. I'm careful not to say negative things about my body. I don't describe others as fat or ugly. I talk about people's differences and talents. We never discuss which foods are fattening or low fat. We talk about proteins, vitamins, minerals, carbohydrates, energy, and food's ability to keep us healthy. My daughter still moves with joy and abandon. I am grateful for every day she's free of body judgements. At almost eight, we've got a good start.

I spoke too soon. I was in the store the other day with my little girl. She tried on a tutu to see how pretty she looked. As she stood there in the lycra body suit, she commented about how fat her stomach was. My heart sank. It has begun.

I want us to teach young girls not to hate themselves. When those curves pop out and girls discover they are different from the boys who seem stronger, braver, and tougher, they start to hate that they're girls. They quit speaking their opinions and ideas. They worry about being liked, not heard. They'd rather be accepted than different. They struggle to fit into tiny bodies and are ashamed when they can't. There is something cruel in messages that strip away our daughters' confidence. And as adult women, we know how hard we have to work to undo the damage.

I am grateful to every person who joins this effort to make peace with our bodies, Together, we are helping to create a new climate of acceptance for women of all ages and body sizes. Already, I am noticing more plus-size models, more choices in larger clothing, and more large women on television, in the magazines, and in the movies. There must be lots of people who are fed up with a culture that adores thinness. Evidently, our voices are more powerful than we realize.

There may be metabolic issues regarding the balance of and the quality of nutrients in dietary intake and weight control that we do not yet understand.[86]

This shift in perspective may take a while. I have better days and less better days. But life is a prayer. It is sacred. I only have a short time to be alive on this planet. Squeezing myself into the "right package" will not be the focus of my life. There is too much that needs doing. There is too much out of balance. There are too many people hurting. So, I dedicate myself to figuring out how I can make things better—for me, for those I care about, and for the world of which I am blessed to be a part. Coming to this peace is the real journey.

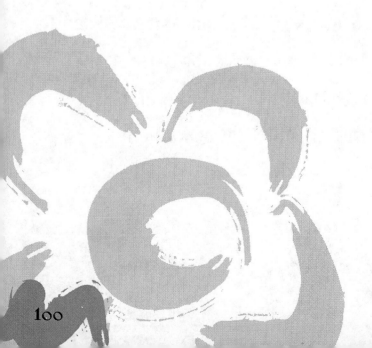

100

Part 3

Women's Prayers, Poems, & Affirmations: Poetry of the Soul

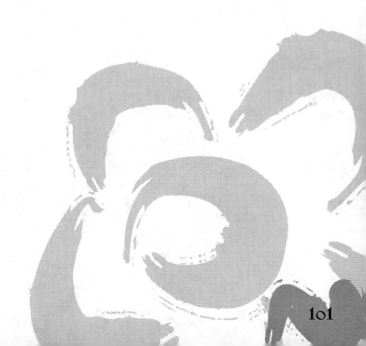

Note: The following affirmations, prayers, poems, and gentle thoughts are for you to use and enjoy in whatever way most helps your own process of coming to peace with your body. May they be an inspiration for you to write
your own promises, affirmations, and love letters to the faithful and wonderful body that carries you through this mysterious, challenging, and most miraculous journey of life.

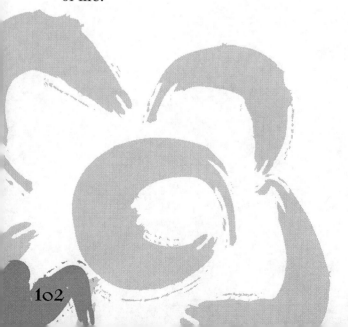

As My Soul Leads Me

Oh, my beloved soul, I acknowledge you this day.

Please lead me this year as I seek to change.

I am growing. I do not know exactly where I am going, but I cherish your support.

I promise to listen as you tell me what you need.

I cannot promise to always follow your directions perfectly, for I often get scared. But I will try.

And I am learning to trust that where you lead me is where I need to be.

I am coming to believe that I have the strength to make a new life for myself. That my courage will not fail me.

I will get tired, but I will find ways to replenish my inner reserve so that I can continue on our journey.

Please send me other souls who will support me along the way so that it does not always feel so solitary.

And please send me clues that tell me I am on the right road. I need them once in awhile.

I will look for your quiet light, sense your gentle voice, and feel your loving touch.

Most of all, remain with me close to my heart. I will hold fast to you throughout every storm and every peaceful season, and rest in your arms each night.

A Promise For Myself

With each new day, I will wake and grow anew.

I will feed myself lovingly, all the things I need.

I will stop and sense the mystery in the moon, trees, earth, and waters around me.

I will forgive myself whenever I do something I wish I hadn't, for I am learning.

I will add more music, color, and movement to my life.

I will keep myself clean and fresh by choosing healthy routines. I will seek to learn more about myself and life from every movie I see, book I read, conversation I hear, or situation I experience.

I will listen to what I am feeling every day, all day long.

I will take time to be silent for a few minutes every day.

I will show those I care for that I am here for them.

I will ask for help when I need it.

I will honor my body when it is hungry and feed it what it needs--whether it is food or something else.

I will face each feeling as it comes. It is part of me, natural, and essential for me to hear.

I will stand firm in my commitment to grow, even when my courage falters.

I will find my own path. Even if I listen for clues from others, I will make my own way in the world.

I will nourish myself in many ways.

I will fill my body with healthy foods eaten with gentleness.

I will move each day to help my energy flow.

I will choose to have supportive people around me.

I will remove myself from unhealthy and unsupportive individuals and circumstances as soon as possible.

I will keep myself open to connect more and more with my sense of a higher power.

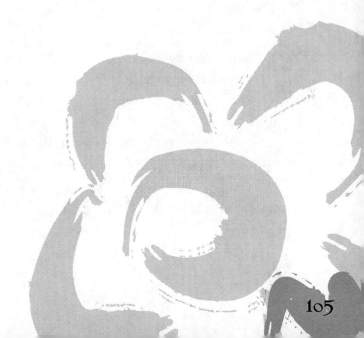

Prayer for the New Year

As I make my way this year through my growth, may I always remember to listen to my deepest self. There, I find my truth, however gentle or harsh it may be.

I am grateful for the courage I have had this past year because it has taken me through dark days and long nights. I have come through each difficult period a little more whole and conscious of who I am and where I have come from.

I hear the voices of my grandmothers and ancestors guiding my footsteps. They gave birth to me through my parents who learned their truths and their weaknesses from them. I hold these truths in my heart and still struggle with these weaknesses.

I hope to better my world just a tiny bit as I pass through it. Whether my mark is big or small, I do not yet know. I seek first and foremost to be as true to myself as I can be, and hope that this positively impacts the earth and her peoples.

Most of all, I practice using my voice. This has been the hardest to learn because it requires that I speak only truth. I am not strong enough to dare to say all that I know all
of the time. I fear hurting others and being hurt in return. But I know my creativity is harnessed to my self-

expression. If I remain mute, I cannot make a contribution of any kind.

I vow to support the people I love. Like a carefully tended garden, I listen to their needs, share my feelings, and watch them grow alongside me. I am no longer sure what to expect from them. I am only just learning what to expect from me.

Last of all, I turn my heart, mind, soul, and body to a perspective larger than mine. I listen, hoping to hear the heartbeat of creation. I wait for the breath of the world on my face each morning to bless me. I puzzle, as always, with the mysteries of why things are as beautifully orchestrated and painfully cruel as they are. With each experience, I get wiser. And with each discovery, I am yet a smaller part of a bigger whole. I only pray that I can remain open to take it all in.

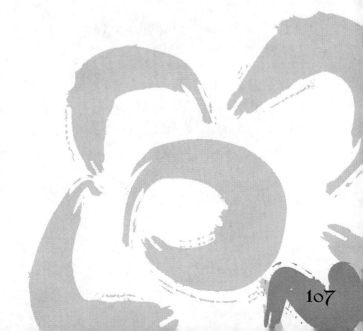

My Promise

I promise to be there for you when you need me—not just when it is convenient.

I promise to listen with all of my heart—and with my story set aside for the moment.

I promise to be open and hear you without judging, for I cannot know the exact path you have chosen or the lesson you are learning.

I promise to accept what you have said and not belittle its meaning by telling you that others have had it worse.

I promise not to laugh at you and suggest that what you are dealing with is trite or silly in some way.

I promise to be as truthful as you want me to be. I can only share my perspective which has been shaped by my own experience and pain.

I promise to acknowledge that we are all on a journey together, growing wiser with each challenge.

I promise to give you space to share your emotions—especially those which you have had to hide such as fear, rage, confusion, doubt, shame, anger, frustration, and guilt.

I promise to be here tomorrow. I will not leave because you tell me things that are hard to hear or to believe.

I promise to be patient when you are struggling with a deeply-rooted demon. We all heal in our own time.

I promise to reach out in case you cannot always ask for what you need. I will create a space of safety to the best of my ability.

I promise to love you as a friend of my soul. No matter how long or short our interaction is, we will remain connected throughout eternity.

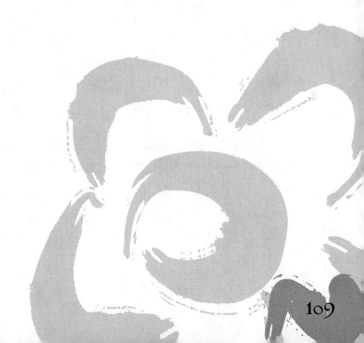

I Resolve

I Resolve to live this year fully, to grow to the best of my capability.

I Resolve to accept my own pace, to know that I step forward slowly, and sometimes even move backwards for a pace or two.

I Resolve to trust my own needs, to know that they guide me and will tell me when I am pushing too hard or when I am doing something to please someone else instead of me.

I Resolve to be kind to myself this year. I know t hat I need gentleness and acceptance for all of my imperfections as well as my abilities.

I Resolve to be more of me even if others might be surprised. I will let my uniqueness out in little ways whether it be through my words, my appearance, my actions, or
my feelings.

I Resolve to pay more attention to my body, to listen when it is hurting, and to try and figure out why.

I Resolve to pay more attention to my feelings, to listen to them when I am hurting and to try and figure out why.

I Resolve to lean on others, to find people I trust even if only a little. This will lighten my load.

I Resolve to remain open to possibilities because life is a surprise. I do not know what is coming. I will rise to meet every challenge and smile at every simple gift life gives me.

I Resolve to hope fiercely for everything I desire. I will keep my dreams alive knowing they lead me into more of me. They give me something to reach for, a purpose.

I Resolve to trust the Universe, the God that made things, the Inner Spirit or Higher Self—I am learning to know there is something bigger than me that I can draw upon for strength and perspective, however I choose to name or describe it.

I Resolve to let go of perfection because I will never succeed. Real perfection is acceptance of the imperfect—knowing it is perfectly fine to be imperfect.

I Resolve to honor my life in the highest way possible, to give myself the care I deserve. I will get the rest and exercise I need; I will create time to play; I will avoid overworking and overpleasing; and I will seek out supportive resources to help me as I grow this year.

I Resolve to befriend the child in me, to let myself be silly and experimental sometimes. I will keep my eyes open for the magic and wonder that ordinary moments can offer when I least expect it.

I Resolve to seek help when I need it, when I am over my head, or hurting from something that might overwhelm me.

I Resolve to find others who struggle to grow as I do, to culture their friendship with patience and loyalty.

I Resolve to accept that not everyone will understand me or be healthy for me to be around. I may have to say no or disappoint another person, and that may hurt me very much.

I Resolve to believe that I deserve to be happy, even if I can't really feel this yet. I will trust it is true.

I Resolve to keep learning more about myself, to discover what I feel and need so I can grow. I will seek out whatever books, support groups, therapy, friends, and routines that will help this process. I know it is a process: it will not happen overnight.

I Resolve to accept that right now, I use food to help me cope. I know that I am trying to heal my hurts so that food will no longer have to bear the burden of comfort-

Love Letter To My Body

I cannot know how hard it is to be responsible for me all day every day. You take me and carry me wherever I want to go. When I get up, you get up. When I want to keep pushing, even though you are tired, you keep going.

Whatever I do to you, you figure out how to make it work for me. If I don't feed you properly, you still give me energy. If I don't sleep enough, you wake up anyway. If I don't get you out in the fresh air, moving and flexing, you never refuse me.

Even if I take you into polluted cities, stuffy offices, and smoke-filled restaurants, you keep breathing. Even if I only have time for fast-food, sugary treats, and no fresh vegetables, you still give me new energy. Even if I race around under stressful deadlines and jammed schedules, you keep up with me. I have never experienced faithfulness so concrete.

I often take you for granted, and I apologize. When you finally react to my abuse by getting sick or collapsing with fatigue, I realize that you, too, need loving attention. You have needs that deserve recognition.

I become more sensitive to your voice each time you demonstrate that you are not indefatigable or infallible. I practice honoring your requests for regular nourishment and rest. I sense your pleasure as I keep you clean, scented, and soft.

As your needs become more clear to me, I struggle with my deepest biases and callous judgements. I struggle to see you as beautiful in every way. I know you dislike my judgement of your various shapes. You cringe when I call a part of you fat. You feel my rejection deeply. You know my shame intimately. Years of diets and hateful thinking have gotten that message home. Your hurt silently filters through every pore.

My judgement mimics the abusive judgements I feel from the social programming around me. For years, I have accepted the standards unconsciously and judged you harshly because of them. As I struggle to get more conscious, I release their fierce grip with each new realization. Yet I am not free. I do not always honor my need to eat. I edit my desire for food. I monitor and measure the growth of each curve as it pushes against my clothes. I look in the mirror and wonder who would truly celebrate the curves of this body with me?

I am grateful that your strength keeps me going as I learn about myself. Your patience during every crazy phase has enabled me to grow, broadening my perspectives and strengthening my values. This slow and labored path is bringing me back to appreciate you.

I am thrilled to have you carry me through each day. I tuck you in lovingly with me each night and listen for what you need from me. Would it have been better for you if I had done something different (how I ate, how I reacted to stress, how much I did, or when I stopped)? Do you need something from me now?

Each loving act I do for you comes back to me. I can feel you relax as I oil my feet or dab flowered scent on my neck. You unwind and float to healing music and light. You revive when I lovingly serve you whole, healthy food.

You are my partner. I learn from you about myself. I learn about my pace. I learn about nurturing and neglect. I learn to recognize nonverbal cues and respond.

I pledge to keep practicing. I can only heal as you heal. So I vow to continue supporting you each day in a way that will allow my full energy, creativity, and hope to come alive. As you faithfully carry my mind, heart, and spirit, I embrace your will to live with quality.

Celebrating Curves

Curves, beautiful, bountiful, spacious curves.

Undulating, rippling, rolling curves.

Round, ripe, comforting curves.

Mature, womanly, and motherly curves.

Staunch, strong, steady curves.

Blessed, holy, sacred, and mysterious curves.

Open, mindful curves.

Willing to go there curves.

Willing to feel it curves.

Willing to taste it curves.

Willing to own it curves.

Overwhelmed and scared curves.

Crunched and panicked curves.

Keep on and we'll make it curves.

Around the corner and we're almost there curves.

Who knows what's out there curves.

There must be more curves.

Questioning, exploring, daring, and finding curves.

Asking, reminding, learning, and growing curves.

We know it's ok curves.

We are people, too, curves.

We love the same curves.

But we look different curves.

No more magazine images curves.

Can't buy into it anymore curves.

Too crazy for me curves.

I sit on the earth curves.

Big round life-giving mother curves.

Got to find my own way curves.

Part of a new way curves.

Honoring me curves.

As I am curves.

For always and always curves.

A woman curves.

A human curves.

A divine being curves.

Under God and celebrating Her curves.

Who am I curves.

A great big beautiful being with curves.

Big Hip Lament

I stand in front of a mirror and strip
and find myself confronted by hips
that ripple and wiggle and push out wide
no matter the clothes they do not hide

the width, the wild unfettered pace
my hips have taken with quite some haste
after having eaten only a few
small things I barely chewed

now they must squeeze into suits so bare
that I shudder to imagine how others will stare
at the size of these thighs and the might they show
in spite of my efforts to keep control

of the calories or is it the fat count now
or the ratio of protein to carbos somehow
that dictates the pattern these hips will take
or is it just genetics that creates the shape

I carry through life that gave me strength
to get a baby out and go to enormous lengths
to balance my life and keep healthy too
while loving my girl, my work, (and me, too)

it's not easy, this effort to be alive
aware, dreaming, and still thrive,
if my hips must suffer a few extra curves
because all my effort goes to how I learn

rather than pleasing the mirror, then so be it
hopefully this will be the way women knit
the pieces of living into a scheme
that honors their hearts, souls...especially their dreams

instead of these hips and fitting them in
to a tiny little suit in which they won't even swim
for fear they might show a part of their rear
in a unflattering position making others sneer

on and on it goes until we resist
and find a new beauty that truly fits
women's bodies, talents, souls, & contributions
to the world by creating wondrous solutions

because of the size of these mighty hips
that hold the power to move and rip
out the wrongs and put forth new connections
that will create a world that honors the feminine

the gentler, the loving, the support of each other
the consideration of all instead of just dollars
the long term well-being of people and earth
to ensure this will work for those yet unbirthed

by loving our hips instead of a mission
to compare, stack, and judge each citizen
for their size, color, money, job, or religion,
neighborhood, accent, homeland, and other differences

better to accept and respect us all
hip size won't matter when we are called
to live as if it counts that we are here
to do the best we can and build from there

Middle Age, Mamas & Peri-Menopause

Once I could fit into jeans that were slim
Though I never qualified as tiny or trim
But my back was smooth and my waist well-defined,
Even though I was blessed with a big behind.

I remember those days and remember I hated
The body I was given for the shapes it created
Hips that bulged, thighs that were ample,
Knees that bent inward and didn't follow the example

Of the pictures that filled magazines and movies
The anchors and hosts of television who we
Saw everyday looking pretty and perfect
Creating the standard that caused each little defect

To magnify and testify in front of my mirror
That I indeed had not conquered my horror
The folds of my body and the shapes that it took
In fact, I found it difficult even to look

At myself with appreciation until I learned how
this obsession with thinness is cruel to us now
So I set out to change how I viewed women's bodies
And discovered mine fit in quite natural boundaries

That were beautiful in their own right
That the words fat, ugly, unattractive & lazy quite
possibly were judgements to keep women worrying
and scurrying to fit instead of contributing

Talents and wit to better this world
Because they were nullified by messages galore
Stating we're not pretty unless we're size four.
Well I changed how I felt and resisted the craze

And found I could actually accept my body's ways.
That is...until I had a baby.
And then my mother's body, her mother's and her moth-
er's too, popped out into sizes I never knew

Ripples of flesh, bellies and folds,
That defy best efforts to get a hold
and return to the body I knew all those years
over which I had shed multiple tears

Which I now would be grateful to see anyhow
compared to the one which reflects back to me now
double chins and soft neck, arms that do sway
and from top to the bottom, a torso with layers.

Who is this that stares back looking so grim
With gray hairs and little lines near the chin
Hands once smooth now starting to show
Deeper lines that prove early youth's on the go

Bigger boobs, thicker waist, and a belly to boot
A matron, a mama, a middle-aged look
That I can't quite get used to and shouldn't accept
According to messages out there and yet

This is how bodies settle into the years.
They get sturdier and stronger to handle the tears
That come with living and making it through
The balancing act and discovering who

We are in our souls and not just appearance.
Trying again to come to a peace, a place
Of acceptance for the body I was given to use
On this journey for wisdom and not just to amuse

No more games to look like I'm thin, in control.
Since diets don't work and my body has slowed
Metabolism and hormones don't seem to know
How to burn up the food that I put in my mouth

Not excessive, just ordinary, yet too much to handle
It stores it and saves it in case I might need
Some extra to sustain me and let me feed
Off my body when the food is all gone.

But this kind effort is all gone to waste
In an era when food is all over the place
Cheap, ready, quick, and yummy
I don't have to wait anymore if I'm hungry

And hungry I've been while raising this kid
I adore yet who's challenged me like none before
To grow, handle, cope, and rise above
Circumstances, boundaries, while feeling love

I've been tired, drained, overly strained
So I've fed the machine that keeps pulling the train
of my life. Yet it seems to need something
other than what I feed it each day.

There is something amiss. For hunger never strays.
This fuel cannot sleep. This food is not time.
These meals do not figure out bills and meet deadlines.
But I use them to help me do all that and more

Because I need to be strong; I have to endure.
So in goes the carbos and protein and vegies
Whole grains and fruit even goodies sometimes
And out come the push of my life keeping time

And my body promises to keep me alive
By sensing the danger, preparing reserves
To weather the panic, the stress, each case of nerves
It captures those calories, stores them away

To help me along on some rainy day.
Still my body keeps slowing while the moon
tides each month go slightly awry signaling soon
ebbing estrogen will throw me a loop.

Have to be tough, I'm told, to be both Mom and dad
to my daughter while creating a life I never had
safe and creative, nurturing and sublime
yet the life muscle to do this challenges my mind

And apparently my body.

I say thanks for carrying me through all these days
While I grow and learn more wisdom in subtler ways
I pledge to keep moving, to sleep, to feed
in multiple ways and we'll see where this leads

Since the dance of the chemicals changing inside
coincides with extraordinary challenges of life,
I must learn to handle a new level of right,
A new way of being—maybe lighter

Than the years so far. But maybe not.
We'll see where it settles. Meanwhile I've got
a healthy—if not skinny—dependable body
that sticks to me faithfully and solidly

No matter what I put it through.
I give it my care, affection, and attention, too
To last through to the end—together and in health.
Making very minor the wish to be svelte.

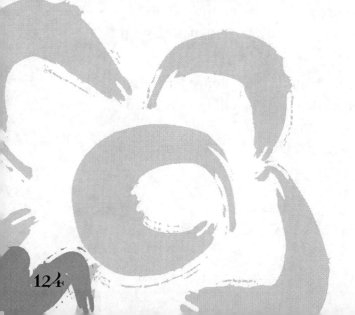

Ode To Chocolate

I leave you sweetest friend, although you fill my soul.

For years, your faithful companionship has been with me through all the hard moments of my life

and the happy ones

and the ordinary, bored ones

and the frustrated, lonely ones

and the completely enraged I don't know what to do ones.

The thought of being without your steady companionship terrifies my heart.

But my body cries out for a rest. No more adrenaline rushes. No more late night jitters.

And so I leave you. I leave your milky, gentle touch.

Yes, separate we must. I need to stand on my own two feet, to find my center without you. To be courageous. To be clean.

Everyday, I grieve. I find only emptiness where you used to be. Nothing can take your place. And I am alone.

But this is right. On my own, at the center of my self, unadorned, I settle down. I listen. I sense. I release. And I grow. On my own terms. Finally.

Abuse

I.

Out of the darkness he comes.

Huge.

Assuming.

Sweet pretties on

hot breath.

Big hands cover me.

Pushes, opens, roars.

Too big, too heavy.

A scream. . .

but no one hears the silence.

Drowning, frantic, trapped,

I wait.

Behind chairs. In closets.

Lost, unfound.

Forever never, never again.

My hair chopped short as ammunition.

With layers of cookies and

cereal, pancakes, noodles and milk.

Can't find pretty here!

How dare you shatter the

raindrops and leave fear

howling through my soul.

Gaping holes hover precariously

near to where I have tread

these past years.

But I found the edge again.

Your footsteps haunt my house

as it shivers with the cold.

I defend my little one's edges.

Through laundry, driving, conversation,

meal-making, I listen fiercely.

Remember to fight, I whisper.

Shout, carry on, never give in.

And always, always tell.

My blood is yours and that of all women.

Those who are given and taken in vain.

Shaken but standing.

Stripped but not stopped.

Mending ourselves one blade, one breath at a time.

Awakening

Snow lies deep, piling high on winter fences.
Tucked inside, the view is quiet, unbroken.
Tracks pattern the fields and skies gray
over my head.

Silence blankets the rooms I walk everyday
Pulling me into doubts, regrets, and wonderings
Insides slide and slip past remembered pathways
overgrown.

Branches naked to the cold, cold sky,
A few leaves yet hang unwilling to drop.
Blown by the howling winter, they fight to remain
claiming the emptied canopy.

My dog knows the truth. Nosing wildly through
snowbanks following a chippy's tunnel, she
declares that winter forces life to underground
without abandon.

So late, I dive into the fiercer places deep,
Locked tight and sealed with relish.
Brandishing search lights, probes, pick axes
fossils appear at every turn.

Each treasure examined, turned, caressed
Until it crumbles in hand. What does it say?
More than a name, a past, a perspective,
mystery awakens.

One small breath in the mighty tide. I want so
much more. Waves rushing, flooding, pulling
me on. Unbalanced, struggling and almost lost...
then I float.

Above, sun simple. Gallant blue giant godfull sky.

I try not. I smile not. I am not. I think not.
Just motion on motion, carrying heartbeat and hope
in an open day.

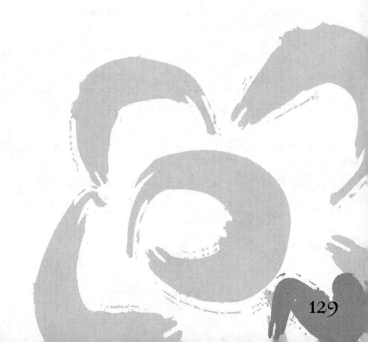

Thank You Body

Thank you hips for carrying me forward this morning.

Thank you legs for being strong enough to push on through the distance I choose to go.

Thank you feet for holding me, lifting me, supporting my every step.

Thank you ribs for sheltering my precious lungs.

Thank you lungs for taking in the sun-filled morning air.

Thank you arms for embracing my life, for grabbing onto what is important to me.

Thank you face for feeling the wind and the sweetness of the day.

Thank you eyes for taking it all in, for keeping me centered, grounded, and here today.

Thank you brain for coordinating this amazing journey.

Thank you fingers for being able to stroke my child's back, fingers, face, hair...

Thank you mouth for swallowing my morning tea.

Thank you heart for being so dedicated, so loyal, so loving.

Thank you soul for wanting so much more.

Thank you stomach for sorting out all that I put in, good and bad.

Thank you intestines for clearing out all that I do not need.

Thank you endocrine system for keeping me balanced, healthy, alive.

Thank you skin for containing me in one miraculous package.

Thank you hair for blowing free and helping me to dream.

Thank you neck for keeping all the communications in my life flowing.

Thank you womb for making me creative, life-producing, feminine, changing, growing.

Thank you teeth for enabling me to bite off what I like and growl at what I don't.

Thank you ears for listening to the higher voice.

Thank you tongue for helping me to sing.

This is my body beautiful today and always.

A New World Fable

Once upon a time, there was a society of women.
Wonderful, warm-hearted women. Strong, capable, leaders of men. Cheerful of soul. Tireless of body. Mothers to
children. An inspiration to all. Each evening these
women gathered to thank the moon which gave the tides.
They
celebrated the ground under their feet which nourished
their people richly. They whispered to the wind which
fed their power and gave them courage to be. And they
fell asleep content.

These women awoke each morning with freshened air
and tickled little ones awake. Filling pots with water and
porridge, the day began with praise to the new light and
another chance to walk the earth. This is the way it had
always been. This is the way they would keep it. Their
partners honored their ways with respect and great
affection. And the elders were greatly proud.

When trouble found these women, as of course it did,
they faced it square on. Sickness, hunger, cold or heat,
anger, and big fear all came in time. They stood as great
ones thinking deeply, listening openly, asking freely,
trusting the river of time and faith. Creation provided
even amidst its endless rhythm of birth and rebirth.
Endings came as crossings-over to new and better ways.

That is not to say that grief did not run deep at the loss of
a child, parent, love, partner, home, or way of life. But
faith had carried them through, and those before. All
they knew had been handed down, bettered, deepened,
and made more whole. Their lives were circles. Great

circles of love. An endless flow of giving easily just as one breathes. In and out. Never thinking. Taking bounty from the Great All and giving back again in honor.

These women were seeds. Each growing tall and true in its own soil: blooming, bearing fruit, and then returning back to enrich the rooting soil which now sustained their offspring. There was nothing better. Nothing more imaginable. Harmony was their way, and it was good.

These women live among us still. Tall, true, silent, listening, they stand nearby. Invisible warriors, they encourage us to remain strong in the face of our own trials. We live in a time without honor for women, without grace for men, and without comfort for children. Freeways, deadlines, newscasts, and obligations replace ancient rhythms. Today, women do not greet each morning with gratitude and close the day with celebration and prayer. We have forgotten the power of our touch to heal, the quieting of our presence, the comfort of a smile given freely. Yet our hearts still carry these ways inside them.

If we listen for guidance, encouragement is there: To gather our souls. To listen to what matters and act upon it. To be anchors for what is right. To light the way for children. To stand in the greatness of simplicity. To honor life's fullness. To greet each day and night with reverence, for it belongs to a much bigger Circle. To simply be as life moves through those we love. We are part of Time, the great tapestry woven every day. This is our legacy. To carry on creatively in strength and great gentility, remaking the world, bettering us all.

The Battlefield Within

Grassy slopes spread out and away. My ancestors have walked here. Their blood streams out through the branches of trees; they fed the soil. Today, I stand not hearing them, not knowing their struggles, just mine.

As a woman I live in another war. Alive in my heart, I cannot breathe in these waters. They bind me and keep me from knowing my role, from knowing myself and why I need to be here now. Why did I come to this earth? Why did I choose to feel all of this pain? Why does this seem so impossible?

I stand at attention, ears peeled wide to catch the inner tick of my heart. I do not want to miss the messenger who comes always with surprise. Whose voice was that? Mine? God's? Angels? Do I listen?

How can I know the truth? This heart of mine feels faint, feeble. It has opened and shut too many times. No more vulnerability. Easier to shut down, die. But the pulse keeps coming. And it grows stronger. The rage behind it pushes through and refuses to be stopped.

No, I will hear it. I will listen to the righteous. I may be unaccompanied, but this path I must tread.

I begin to march. Not much to support me, yet I keep on. The rolling fields greet me and invite me to continue. The hills rise up and testify that there is a majesty to my purpose. I see before me a ribbon of river deep, wide, shimmering. Imperceptibly moving. Undercurrents carrying everything forward.

I, too, am a river running to my ocean. To laughingly greet the great mother sea. To sit at her feet before merging into the larger pulse that moves us all.

Today, I do not know if I am on the right path. The underbrush is thick and my progress is slow. I feel grateful to see a place where others have passed before. I feel less alone.

I could always retreat but it doesn't make sense. How can I turn back? Nothing will ever be the same again. I keep going.

I find a hill at sunset. I watch the light dim and spread out in blankets of orange and dusky pinks. My heart is soothed. I usher it into my inner chamber and hold on tight. I do not want this feeling to end. The arms of my purpose are around me. Everywhere are beating hearts, whispering souls that move me to continue the battle. To move forward into history. To fight for humane answers to how we must live.

I stand in the long line of women, silent, unable to speak their hearts' truth. Powerless to take the reins. We are new to this rabble-rousing courage it takes to keep going. It is awkward and uncomfortable most of the time.

We want to stand before men that honor our differences,

that greet us as equals, that concede to violence, and use their warrior hearts for nurturing us all. We are their mothers, partners, lovers, and sisters. We ask them to come with us.

But first we must walk our own road. To gain unshakable strength. We move, bend, and flow across our terrain. A silent power growing from one first small trickle. Gathering streams of experience, our capacity grows. We will get to that sea, and we will be strong.

And so I take another step and will take another again tomorrow. I pledge my allegiance to my original cause. And I step forward again.

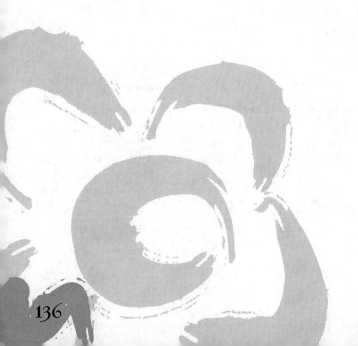

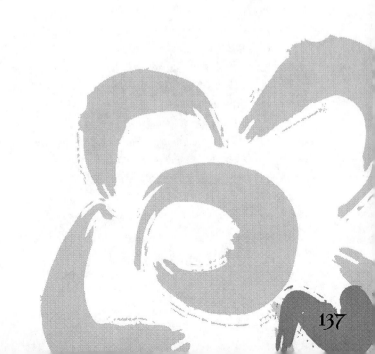

Source Notes

1   Christiane Northrup, <u>Women's Bodies, Women's Wisdom</u>

2   <u>Star Tribune</u>, June 1, 1994

3   Carolyn Costin, <u>Our Dieting Daughters</u>

4   <u>USA Weekend</u>, Feb 20-22, 1998

5   National Institute of Mental Health

6   National Center for Health Statistics; National Institute of Mental Health

7   National Institute of Mental Health

8   New Moon Network, "Eating Disorders in Girl Athletes," Jul/Aug 1995

9   <u>Weight Watchers Magazine</u>, July, 1991

10 <u>New Moon</u>, "Body Language: Kathy Rigby on Girls' Athletes Eating
        Disorders, Jul/Aug, 1995

11 <u>Journal of Abnormal Psychology</u>

12 <u>Essence</u>, January 1994, "Dangerous Eating""

13 Mimi & Mark Nichter and Sheila Parker, University of Arizona

14 Loretta DiPietro, PhD, Assistant Professor of Epidemiology,
        Yale University

15 <u>Ar'n't I a Woman</u>, "The Life Cycle of a Female Slave"

16 Corynne Corbett, Editor, <u>MODE Magazine</u>

17 World News Tonight, 1998

18 <u>Teen People</u>, "Weighty Issues," Nov,1998

19 Esther Rothblum, PhD, University of Vermont

20 Colleen Rand, PhD, University of Florida

21 <u>Losing It: America's Obession with Weight and the Industry that Feeds
        on it</u>, Laura Fraser

22 Sharlene Hesse-Biber, PhD, <u>Eating Patterns & Eating Disorders Among
        Boston College Students</u>, March, 1988

23 Melissa Lavitt, Associate Professor, Social Work, Arizona State University

24 Howard Green, Spokesperson, Walt Disney Pictures, May, 1995

25 Linda Valdez, <u>Arizona Republic</u>, May, 1995

26 <u>Marie Clair</u>, January, 1998

27 Katherine Phillips, MD, <u>The Broken Mirror</u>

28 Sharlene Hesse-Biber, PhD, <u>Eating Patterns & Eating Disorders Among
        Boston College Students</u>, March, 1988

29 *"Fitness for EveryBody," Sweatshop News, St Paul, MN, Apr-Jun, 1998*

30 *Health Line, Murray State University*

31 *Mimi Nichter, <u>Fat Talk</u>*

32 *<u>International Journal of Sports Medicine</u> , 1989*

33 *<u>Journal of Obesity and Weight Regulations</u>, 1984*

34 *<u>Losing It: America's Obession with Weight and the Industry that Feeds</u>
      <u>on it</u>, Laura Fraser*

35 *Xavier Pi-Sunyer, MD, New York St. Luke's Hospital*

36 *Kelly Brownell, Yale University*

37 *Leah Graves, RD, LD, 1988 National Eating Disorders Screening Program*

38 *Shannon Daley, PhD, "Dealing with Depression," <u>Teen People</u>, Oct, 1998*

39 *Dr. Susan Yanovski, National Institutes of Health*

40 *Harvard School of Public Health*

41 *Network for Size Esteem, "International No Diet Day Food for Thought"*

42 *<u>Life Magazine</u>, "Do I Look Fat to You?," February, 1995*

43 *Gallop Poll, Summer, 1995*

44 *Adrienne Ressler, Introductory Remarks, 3rd Annual Renfrew Conference*

45 *<u>Eating Well</u>, "Kids at the Crossroads," Sept-Oct, 1995*

46 *Nicki Crick, Assistant Professor, University of Illinois at
      Urbana-Champaign*

47 *<u>Girl</u>, "Tips for Killer Confidence," Fall, 1998*

48 *<u>Star</u>, "Hollywood's Deadly Obsession With Losing Weight," Oct. 27, 1998*

49 *<u>People</u>, "Who Says Size Counts," September 29, 1997*

50 *Patricia Weenolsen, PhD, University of California--Santa Cruz*

51 *Thomas O'Guinn, PhD, Associate Professor of Advertising, University of
      Illinois*

52 *Daniel Perlman, PhD, School of Family and Nutritional Sciences,
      University of British Columbia--Vancouver*

53 *Carol Sheinkopf, CSW, New York, NY*

54 *Thomas Patrick Malone, MD and Patrick Thomas Malone, MD,
      <u>The Art of Intimacy</u>*

55 *<u>Madmoiselle</u>, "Anatomy of a Loser," October, 1988*

56 *Nancy Friday, <u>Jealousy</u>*

57 Glamour, "Jealousy, Success, and Self-Esteem," September, 1985

58 BBW, "Food & Women," Jun, 1991

59 Susan Basow, PhD, Associate Professor of Psychology, Lafayette College

60 Henry Jaglom, Producer & Director, Eating (film)

61 Eating (film)

62 Gone With the Wind (film)

63 Glamour, "Learning to Blow"

64 New York Times, "Women's Success: A Darker Side," Sept 10, 1986

65 Barbara Sternberg, Consultant, Weight Watchers International, 1986

66 Hillel Schwartz, Never Satisfied: a Cultural History of Diets,
       Fantasies & Fat

67 Trish Ratto, RD, Health Promotion, Cowell Hospital, Berkeley

68 Fima Lifshz, MD, Professor of Pediatrics, Cornell University
       Medical College

69 Michael Pugliese, MD, et al, Pediatrics, "Parental Health Beliefs as
       a Cause of Nonorganic Failure to Thrive," Aug 1987

70 Laurel Mellin, RD, Clinical Professor of Pediatrics and Director, Center
       for Adolescent Obesity, University of California--San Francisco

71 Medical Self Care, "Fear of Fat Goes Fanatic, " Sept/Oct 1988

72 Glamour, "The Pressure to be Perfect," January, 1996

73 Eric Goodman, Instructor, Miami University

74 The Dieter's Dilemma, William Bennett and Joel Gurin

75 MODE, "Art on a Grand Scale," August, 1998

76 Radiance, "When Women Stop Hating Their Bodies," Fall, 1995

77 Vogue, "The Age of Self Control," April, 1987

78 Beauty Bound, Rita Jackaway Freedman, PhD

79 Body Trust: Undieting Your Way to Health & Happiness, Dayle Hayes, MS

80 The Healthy Weight Journal, Frances Berg, Editor,

81 Big Beautiful Women/BBW, "The Fat Gene: Friend or Foe?," Apr, 1995

82 Networker, "Body Politics," Stephen Madigan, PhD, Nov/Dec, 1994

83 New Moon, "How Aggravating," June, 1995

84 Center for Women Policy Studies, 1995

85 The Diet-Free Solution, Laurel Mellin

86 "Learning to Live in Our Bodies," keynote by Rebecca Radcliffe

EASE
Living to
Grow™
Resources

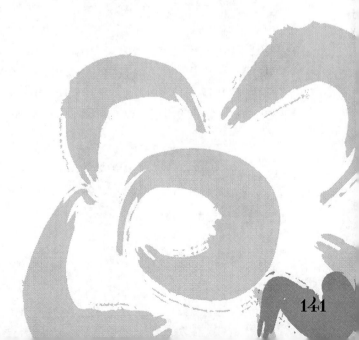

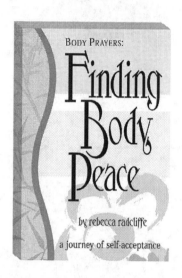

Body Prayers™: Finding Body Peace—A Journey of Self-Acceptance

By Rebecca Radcliffe

***Body Prayers*™** takes the reader through an inner journey about society's obsession with thinness and the harmful effect it has on self-esteem. It helps women of any age come to question society's narrow definition of beauty and find greater self-acceptance for their bodies. Ending on a poetic and inspirational note, ***Body Prayers*™** affirms every woman's right to embrace her unique beauty and to express her talents in the world which so desperately needs feminine perspectives today.

"Soulful, heart-warming, and uplifting.
This is a breath of fresh air!"

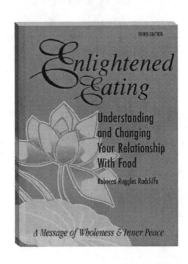

Enlightened Eating™: Understanding and Changing Your Relationship With Food

By Rebecca Radcliffe

Enlightened Eating™ is a personal, compassionate resource for those who struggle with eating issues and feel self-conscious about their bodies. In a deeply insightful, simple, and uniquely understandable way, it explores how stress, eating, and self-esteem are so closely linked, and inspires and encourages us to make healthier life choices. Complete with 34 exercises for making personal change, this book provides much needed insight to heal eating concerns, body hatred, and low self image. *Enlightened Eating™,* with its sections on women's issues, inner spirit, food & feelings, stress, and surviving holidays, is used by individuals, support groups, and counselors nationwide.

> *" This is the best book I've read on the subject!"*

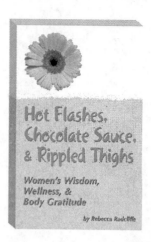

Hot Flashes, Chocolate Sauce, &
Rippled Thighs
Women's Wisdom,
Wellness, &
Body Gratitude
by Rebecca Radcliffe

Hot Flashes, Chocolate Sauce, & Rippled Thighs: Women's Wisdom, Wellness, Self-Acceptance, & Joy

By Rebecca Radcliffe

Hot Flashes, Chocolate Sauce, & Rippled Thighs is a delightful book for adult women who are interested in making peace with their bodies and exploring the process of finding balance and meaning as their lives unfold. *Hot Flashes, Chocolate Sauce, & Rippled Thighs* reminds us that our bodies are sacred and that each stage of life has its purpose. Focusing on women's vitality, *Hot Flashes* encourages women to consider that they may live long, energetic lives. This gives us the opportunity to use our many talents, energy, and values to create richer lives for ourselves and better the world instead of worrying about our dress size..

"This book takes a wonderfully fresh perspective on
the deeper meaning of women's lives."

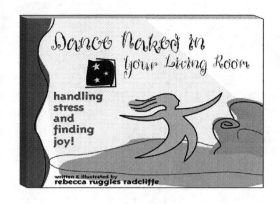

Dance Naked In Your Living Room: Handling Stress & Finding Joy

By Rebecca Radcliffe

Dance Naked In Your Living Room™ is a playful, helpful tool for learning how to cope with stress without turning to food—or any unhealthy pattern. Because learning to handle stress is such an important key to change emotional eating, *Dance Naked*™ helps us learn to nurture and take care of ourselves and find moments of joy in the process. It offers more than 120+ healthy ways to unwind that can be done anywhere, anytime, and without cost. What a great way to be good to yourself and those you care about.

"A delightful answer to the high-pressure stress that plagues us all!"

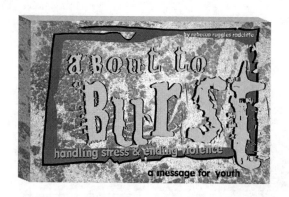

About To Burst™: Handling Stress & Ending Violence—A Message for Youth

by Rebecca Radcliffe

Finally, a great resource for youth under stress! In a chaotic world that leads kids to use eating, aggression, drugs, drinking, sex, and guns as ways to cope with their stress, new solutions are needed desparately. *About To Burst™* is a hip, creative book that helps young people learn to positively deal with the stresses in their lives—without doing harm to themselves or others. *About To Burst™* talks about stress in a way that young people can relate to—and then offers more than 120 creative alternatives for kids to use when pressures at home, school, work, in relationships, or in the environment overwhelm them. This book offers solutions to help prevent violence and self-destructive choices among teens. *About To Burst™* is a helpful tool for parents, educators, counselors, and anyone who cares about young lives.

"A big help for the pressure young people feel

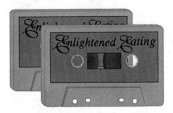

The Enlightened Eating™ Tape Set

is a set of four heart-warming, uplifting, and introductory discussions that will trigger new insights and understanding. Topics include emotional eating, body hatred, eating disorders, and the search for meaning.

" Such a private and easy introduction!"

Developing Healthier Eating Habits

helps anyone with eating issues begin to make positive change. A practical pocket-guide to creating new eating patterns. Excellent handout.

"A great help for students & clients"

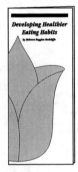

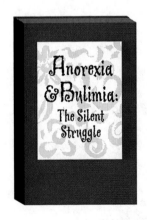

Anorexia & Bulimia: The Silent Struggle

is an intimate and personal video discussion of what eating disorders are, how they affect the body, what causes these problems, what kind of help someone needs, and what friends or family can do to help. For small group or individual viewing. 29 min. A quiet version of Rebecca's popular talk.*

*(No rentals or previews)

" A compassionate introduction to eating disorders and the struggle to recover."

Living to Grow™ Talks:

Presentations For Greater Awareness, Joy, Esteem, Trust, Confidence, & Compassion

by Rebecca Radcliffe

People today feel the pressure of fast-paced lives which leave them vulnerable to stress, low self-esteem, and

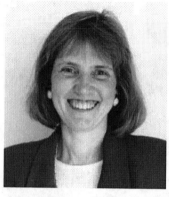

unhealthy choices. All of us need inspiration to discover healthier ways of living. Rebecca's presentations and workshops provide inspiration and encouragement to creatively pursue personal growth and the process of finding joy. This exciting inner journey is both highly individual and amazingly universal.

Sample Topics*

- *Body Prayers™: Finding Body Peace*
- *Learning To Live In Our Bodies: Changing Emotional Eating and Body-Hatred*
- *Dance Naked In Your Living Room: Handling Stress and Finding Joy*
- *Lives in Balance: The Many Choices Toward Wellness*
- *Living To Grow: Choosing To Be Conscious, Courageous, and Creative*
- *Our Inner Spirit: Nourishing Our Souls*
- *About to Burst™: Beyond Violence to Hope*

**Call (800) 470-GROW (4769) or go to
www.rebeccaradcliffe.com for information .**

*For: Keynotes, Workshops, Women's Programs, Wellness Events, Community Education, Awareness Weeks, In-Services, Professional Trainings, Assemblies, Panel Discussions, Retreats, Commencements, Corporate Meetings, Luncheon Lectures, Orientation, Men's Groups, Conferences, Violence Prevention Programs

Order by phone: 1-800-470-4769   fax: 1-720-559-9267
e-mail vial: www.livingtogrow.com Mail: EASE, P.O. Box 8032,
Mpls. MN 55408. Purchase orders accepted.
Sorry, no credit cards at this time.

Order Form

- **Books**
  —Body Prayers™, $17.00
  —Enlightened Eating™, $18.95
  —Dance Naked In Your Living Room, $12.00
  —Hot Flashes™, $17.00
  —About to Burst, $15.00

- **Other Resources**
  —Enlightened Eating™ Tape Series, $19.95
  —Anorexia & Bulimia: The Silent Struggle, $39.95
  — ____ copies of Developing Healthier Eating Habits.*(see chart below)*

Quantity	Price	Quantity	Price
1	2.50	21-35	1.00 ea.
2-9	2.00 ea.	35+	.75 ea.
10-20	1.50 ea.		

- **Mailing List** *(list not sold or shared; mailings usually 1-2 times per year)*

- Please add my name to your mailing list.

- **Shipping & Handling**

For order totals of:	Add:	For order totals of:	Add:
$3.00 to $20.00	$4.00	$81.00 to $100.00	$8.00
$21.00 to $40.00	$5.00	$101.00 to $120.00	$9.00
$41.00 to $60.00	$6.00	$121.00 to $140.00	$10.00
$61.00 to $80.00	$7.00	$141.00 or more... add 8% of your order total	

- | **Order Total $** | U.S. Dollars Only |

— I have enclosed a check made payable to **EASE**™.

PLEASE PRINT CLEARLY:

Name (Individual name required for tracking orders)

Title/Department

Organization

Address (Please use street address for UPS orders)

City   State   Zip

Phone Number (Include for questions about your order)

Email (Include for questions about your order)

Send check and order form to EASE™, P.O. Box 8032, Mpls, MN 55408-0032.
Allow 3-6 weeks for delivery. Thank you! Questions? 1-800-470-4769   23.2BP

Acknowledgements

Once again, my fabulous graphic designer and sister, Beth Ruggles, has created a marvelous design for **Body Prayers**. I could not do what I do without her help. My sweet daughter, Chloe, who appears a few times in this book, is my ever-present inspiration for this attempt to better women's lives.

I also thank two professors of mine: Mark D. Savin, who helped shape my writing, and Michael Dennis Brown, who introduced me to a different way of "seeing" into words.

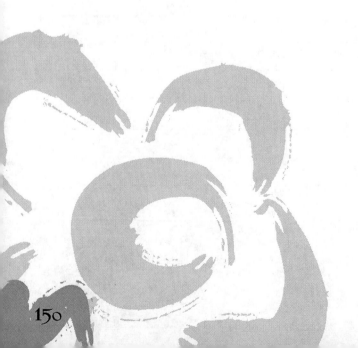

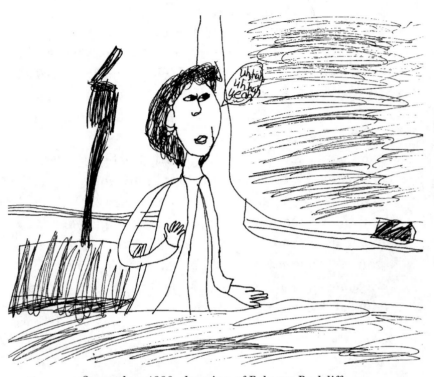

September, 1998, drawing of Rebecca Radcliffe
by author's daughter, Chloe

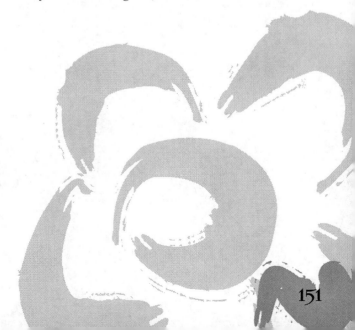

About Rebecca Radcliffe

Rebecca Radcliffe, is author of *Enlightened Eating: Understanding & Changing Your Relationship With Food; Dance Naked In Your Living Room: Handling Stress & Finding Joy; Hot Flashes, Chocolate Sauce, & Rippled Thighs; and About to Burst: Handling Stress & Ending Violence.* She is a national speaker, workshop leader, and expert on stress, growth psychology, women's issues, and life balance with an uplifting and soulful perspective. Rebecca is Executive Director of EASE™ Publications and Resources, an organization dedicated to enhancing personal growth and self-esteem. She speaks frequently nationwide at many universities, communities, schools, health events, national conferences, corporations, retreats, and seminars.